How Doctors Kill

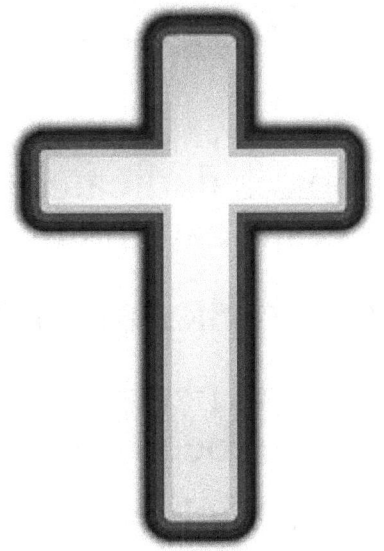

How Angels Die

A LIFE AND DEATH STRUGGLE WITH HOSPITALS, DOCTORS, DECEPTION AND CANCER

A Memoir by Professor Joseph S. Masterson
B.A., J.D., L.L.M.

<u>DEDICATION</u>

This book is dedicated to my granddaughters,

Amanda and Skylar Masterson.

Without their existence in my life, it could not have been written.

It is through them that
The Spirit of Mi Song will be continued.

The author wishes to acknowledge his friend Robert Shookster for the considerable time spent in his revisions and editing of this manuscript.

TABLE OF CONTENTS

TABLE OF CONTENTS (cont.)

INTRODUCTION

This is a book about a remarkable woman by the name of Mi Song. She was not only a friend but she was someone with whom I experienced the suffering of cancer and eventually the meaning of death. It was the death of someone I cared about very much. It is also a book about her struggle in the face of a family who did not understand what was happening to her, did not help her get the best medical advice that she could have obtained and doctors and hospitals that failed her. Doctors and hospitals that I believe, are failing most of the cancer patients today in this country. This is the preface to the book and is simply my feelings about what happened to her. She can no longer speak. She can no longer tell people how she felt about her journey, but I can. I intend to do it in this book.

CHAPTER 1: "THE WOMAN"

Mi Song was born in South Korea on September 16, 1954. South Korea only a few years before suffered under the yoke of the Japanese Imperial Army. The South Korean women were used as concubines for Japanese troops. Their lands were ransacked and their people were mistreated and murdered. This is the backdrop to some of the feelings that she had in her life. Feelings that told her that most good things come only after a struggle. That struggle moreover is sometimes necessary. She was born into a family that had one sister and one brother, both older than she. Her father and mother, although they lived together, lived a rather lower middle class existence.

As she grew up, she was quite exceptional. Her grade school records indicate that she was a high achiever. Even in sports, she seemed to excel and in many instances, outperformed the boys in her grade group. As a matter of fact, her father once commented to her mother that, "she must be a boy." The reader should note that in Asian families, even today, boys are prized over girls but she was the exception. In high school, she also excelled. She was a South Korean National champion swimmer. In fact, she went to the Olympics in the early seventies. She was a top long distance runner and she was beautiful, Very beautiful. She even sang on national South Korean radio and in fact, was at one time considered to be one of the most beautiful women in Asia.

Having accomplished all of this, and being who she was, she decided that she was going to marry an American serviceman, a captain, and the both of them would come to the United States and settle here. And that, they did.

She was not without fault. Mi was very conscious of her exceptional ability. Sometimes she was difficult to deal with. She was emotional and she was passionate. She would tell you exactly what she thought. She pulled no punches and sometimes you might feel insulted by what she had said. Even if she insulted you, it was rare that she would make an apology. She had tremendous self-confidence. She was able to speak four languages and she received a college degree here in the U.S. There was almost nothing she could not accomplish.

How did I know her? Well, I first met her at a lecture that I gave on Abraham Lincoln in the summer of 1997. After the lecture, she came up and introduced herself. I of course was struck with the beauty of the woman in front of me talking about Abraham Lincoln in a South Korean accent. I asked for her card, which she gave to me, and I gave my contact information to her. I didn't hear from her again for some months.

But that is how I met her and I can tell you that as I dictate this book today that I can see her standing in front of me just as clearly as I did see her back in the late 1990's.

Chapter 2: Cancer

I did not hear from her for some time until I received a call, I guess it was in the year 2002, it might have been 2001. It was on my birthday and as soon as I heard the voice on the other end, I of course recognized who it was. I was very happy to hear from her. Especially on my birthday. She didn't know it was my birthday, that's how accidental it all was. She seemed to be troubled. She had a voice that I recall as being quite strong but now seemed timid and fearful. She said I have something to tell you. She said I am reluctant to tell it to you because the friends that I have told it to in the recent past have all left me. She said it's something apparently no one wants to hear and no one wants to help me with. I said "what is it", thinking what could it be? She said, "I have cancer." All I can tell you is that when I heard that and it was on my birthday, July 17, yes, I knew then, I knew that I would be part of this woman's life for as long as she lived or I lived. I assured her that I would not be that kind of friend and asked her to describe exactly what kind of cancer she had. It was breast cancer. I knew very little about cancer at that time. The only thing I knew was that it seemed to always carry a death sentence with it, it was a very difficult disease, and still is.

So, we agreed to meet and we did. I went down to Princeton one Saturday where she was living in a small apartment. She took me out and showed me her new car that she had just purchased and was quite pleased with that. What I didn't know is that as I looked at her and she looked so beautiful to me, what I didn't know was that she had in the last week or two lost almost all of her hair. She was later to tell me that it would come out in clumps in the morning on her bed and she would cry about it. She was wearing a wig and it looked to me to be natural, very well kept. She also told me humorously that a tradesman had delivered something to her door and she forgot to put on the wig and went to the door with a bare head and she said she almost scared the life out of the poor fellow.

We went out to eat lunch and we talked about the meaning of friendship and that her doctor said that she would have to undergo, chemotherapy once or twice a week and then three or four months of radiation. She told me how the cancer was discovered. Not by her doctor who initially told her it was nothing to worry about but rather by her doing a self-examination. It was she who finally convinced the doctor that this was a little bit more than a cyst. She left me that day with the feeling that "we" were going to beat this thing. I can tell you that she had over whelming confidence. She never believed that she could die from cancer.

She looked strong. She had been a national running champion, swimming champion, she was so beautiful. I just couldn't believe that a cell or series of cells operating in her body and operating apparently out of control could take her life. I just couldn't believe it.

Chapter 3:
Treatment And Marriage

And so she went through the chemo and radiation for a couple of months and as we got to know each other better, we decided that we would get engaged. We even planned a marriage for November of 2002. We tried also to help her brother and sister with immigration problems. Apparently they had been told by a Korean businessman that if they paid him $5-10,000 or whatever it was, they could get their green card. But now it was apparent that he was a fraud and that in fact, they were here illegally. We tried to help with that. We tried to get lawyers involved to help them but we were unable to do it. She was here legally. She had come with her army husband and she got a green card. She was safe, but they were not. She was worried about that.

In any event, she went through the chemo and she, before we could marry, sends some of my clothes over to Korea. Her family had to approve of the marriage and they sent the clothes to see how long I had to live (believe it or not) and what kind of personality I would have and whether I would make a good husband. She was somewhat younger than I was. She was only 47 years old and I am not going to give my age but I was much older. That is what apparently had to be done to have the marriage approved. They were told by a fortune teller in Korea that I would have a long life and had a good personality. Boy, he missed that one but that is what they were told and we planned a wedding for November. Without going into detail, that was cancelled until she got stronger and had come out of the cancer experience with no more chemo and no more radiation. Finally, her hair started growing back. The doctors told her that her cancer was in remission.

Soon she and I began to have more personality clashes and it became apparent that we were too much alike to live a life together and so we abandoned out plans for marriage.

She was now apparently healthy with her cancer in remission and working full-time she met another fellow, got engaged and I did not hear from her for approximately a year or a year and a half. Sometime in early 2003 (or a little later than that) I got a telephone call again. All bad news comes through the phone. It was Mi Song on the other end. I was very happy to hear from her. I had not heard from her in a long time. We talked about minor things for a few minutes and then she said I have something to tell you. I need your help. "What is it?" I asked in a hesitant way. "My cancer has returned", she softly replied. Oh God, her cancer it back, I thought. So, I said "what hospital are you with?", and she said, "Robert Wood Johnson". "I have a doctor, Dr. Rishe. He is taking care of me". She told me too that her fiancé was not very helpful. "He is disappointed that I have it", she said sadly. I recalled her telling me sometime before about how she lost her friends when they heard about this kind of a thing. I said to her, of course I would help her thinking that this was bad news. I knew I would do anything I could and she and I now established an even better relationship than we had before. Every time she would have chemotherapy, I would try to go with her. Every time she had radiation or visited a doctor, I would talk to her about it until finally when I realized that she didn't seem to have a grip on exactly how serious this was or exactly how they were going about fixing it, I asked her if I could go with her, and indeed I did.

I went with her for about five or six meetings with Dr. Rishe at Robert Wood Johnson until, believe it or not, Dr. Rishe said to her one day (and he knew I was an attorney), he said to her "if he continues to come to the meetings with you, I'm going to have to recommend that another doctor take over your care". I guess his objections to me were that I would ask questions, I would want to know what her progress was exactly what medicines were being used on her and he didn't like all that. I can tell you that is not unusual. Doctors like to play God. Doctors like you not to know what exactly what they are telling you. They talk in "doctor speak" and unless you have someone with you, you are going to have a really difficult time during your cancer experience. You are a victim, you are afraid, you are terrified. You sometimes hear the words but don't know what you are hearing and that was exactly what was happening to her. Finally, in December of 2003, Dr. Rishe indicated to her that there was nothing more that he could do for her. That her cancer now was so serious that it was not responding to the treatment that he felt would be effective for that cancer and he was discharging her as a patient. Can you believe that? I could not!

CHAPTER 4: BAD DOCTORS

At this point in time, she was engaged to another fellow. Mi was so beautiful it didn't take her long to attract men and she had a new suitor. The one I spoke about previously left because of the cancer. He couldn't handle that. The new suitor, his name was Marvin, was a Professor of computer technology at one of the Universities here in New Jersey. A very nice fellow. He knew of her cancer and was willing to go through the struggle with her. Both he and she called me the night that Dr. Rishe had discharged her and told me what he had said. Now, I don't accept everything doctors tell you. I think everyone should seek a second opinion, perhaps a third, especially when you are talking about something as serious as cancer. So I suggested to her that she allow me two days, I think this was a Tuesday or Wednesday, to allow me to the end of the week to find someone for her to rely upon and give us his opinion and let's see how it coincides or doesn't coincide with Dr. Rishe's opinion.

I received a magazine, called New York Magazine and every year New York Magazine publishes a list of the best doctors in New York with their specialties and what hospital they are affiliated with. I had read about a Dr. Oster who was an oncologist, who was published, who was well respected and New York Magazine almost every year consistently named him as one of the best doctors in New York. I decided I was going to try and get Dr. Oster for her care. Dr. Oster was affiliated Columbia Presbyterian Hospital and I knew something about the hospital because I had been up there about two years earlier with the President of the hospital being interviewed for a General Counsel position. I decided to call the president of the hospital and see if I can get a little pressure put on Dr. Oster if necessary to see Mi Song the following Monday. I called and talked to his secretary and made up a story - and that story was, that I was counsel to Governor McGreevy and Governor McGreevy was interested in Mi Song, because Mi Song's family had contributed significant funds to his election campaign. Well, that did it. The secretary told me that someone would get back to me as soon as possible and within five to ten minutes, the Executive Vice President called me. He asked what doctor do you want to see and I said Dr. Oster. He replied that he would talk to him and that I should have Mi Song there at 9:00 on Monday morning and he would see us.

I hung up and called Mi Song, I told her we have one of the best doctors in the country and we are going to bring you over to Columbia Presbyterian on Monday. I will go with you, I said, and we will have a consultation with Dr. Oster. I can tell you I felt better about that, because I thought that if we were lucky there is a guy out there, a doctor that is humane, who is smart and may have another answer to this problem, or at least give her some hope. Not just discharge her with the feeling there is nothing else that can be done for her. I think that is inhumane and I think it is unprofessional. In any event, Monday morning came and she and I went in to see Dr. Oster.

Oster's office was small. I was somewhat surprised. It was festooned with covers of New York Magazine announcing that he was the doctor of the year or one of the best doctors in New York. Many magazines were pinned to the wall. Finally, Dr. Oster comes in and seemed to be very affable, very friendly, very talkative and he questioned her about her treatment and what the doctors had said about her. We had some of her records that he had seen previously. I said to him, "Dr. Rishe indicates that there is nothing more that can be done for her".

Mi Song is sitting there listening and he said "that is nonsense". "I can reduce that tumor that is on your chest", and he looked at it. She in fact had a tumor that was protruding from the top of her chest, two or three of them. He said, "I will reduce those and eventually get rid of them and you will see a marked reduction within three weeks". Her remark was "thank God, I now have some hope". I can tell you I felt so much better to hear that. So much better to see a doctor confident that he can do something to save her precious life. She asked if she could be excused to go to the bathroom and when she did I said to Dr. Oster, "how is it that someone like Dr. Rishe could tell her nothing more could be done". I said "when can we start?". We set a date within three or four days. She now started treatment with Dr. Oster, but let me go back and give the reader some of my thoughts.

She was treated from the day we found out she had cancer (and including Dr. Oster) badly. It seems to me that doctors don't want anyone to ask questions or question what they have to say about your particular illness and if someone dares to do that, the relationship with the doctor will suffer. I had that problem with Dr. Rishe at Robert Wood Johnson. The problem as I stated before was that I would go to the meetings with her and I can tell you that these doctors talk to patients in "doctor speak" and most of the time one doesn't know what they are saying. I would go to meetings with her and ask questions. I would question results. I would want to see x-rays and her doctors didn't like all of that. They didn't want to do it. As a matter of fact, at one point they were using an experimental drug on her. They didn't tell her about that but she had to sign some kind of a contract. I thought that was truly unusual and something that should not have been done. I told him that.

So it came to the point that Dr. Rishe threatened her. Imagine, a doctor threatening a cancer patient who is quite sick. The threat was if you keep bringing this lawyer with you to the meetings (and she was telling him, he is my best friend and coming as a friend) you are going to have to get another doctor.

CHAPTER 5: BE INFORMED

I must say however, there are many good professional people. I recall one doctor visit when Mi Song needed a biopsy. They put her on a table, deadened her shoulders and her chest and they cut out a little piece of some tissue right above her chest wall where the tumor was. I was with her and held her hand as they were doing this and I could see her starting to cry. A tear in fact fell on my hand. She got off the table and got dressed and as she was walking out of the room the nurse appeared and said to her, "good luck Mi" and threw her arms around her. Both of them started to cry. There are a lot of people who care. There are people who really worry about the patient, but not enough, not enough. Do you know for example, that one-hundred thousand people will die in hospitals this year, this year because these hospitals are negligent? You won't die because of the reason that brought you there, you're going to die because of negligence that exists there. Someone didn't wash their hands, or they let something infect you. This doesn't even take into account the negligence of doctors and how many people die because of that! It is very difficult to get this information. Very difficult.

As a matter of fact when Mi was being treated at Columbia Presbyterian, we found out after she finished her treatments, and I am a little ahead of myself in my story, but we found out that there was legionnaire's disease at the hospital at the time she was there. In the water! The hospital didn't tell anybody that. This is Columbia

Presbyterian Hospital. It is not Jacoby Hospital, which apparently is the worst hospital in the country.

Now Oster has given us a "new lease on life" and I take her home. I had a car ready for her. She sat in the back and as I took her home we both felt that things would now get better for her. I remember her taking some money from her pocket and putting it in my hand. She said I know you have to pay the driver. I remember leaving her house that night and her standing under the light waving goodbye. I remember going home to my own bed and thanking God for Dr. Oster and for a treatment that I was absolutely convinced was going to work. After all, didn't he say that in three weeks we would see a reduction? I was able to sleep.

Well, she started her treatment and I went with her for most of them and Marvin, who was now married to her was going with her for the others. When he couldn't go, I would go. Dr. Oster seemed to be different now. He was less talkative. He would come into the room and spend little time with us. He would look at the large mounds of tissue coming out of her chest now, (the cancer tumors) and just shake his head and say, "I find no bad news in your blood." "There are no cancer markers showing up in your blood and that is good news." He didn't want to take questions and finally after three weeks, she said these tumors are not getting smaller and I'm not feeling better. When we would tell that to Dr. Oster, he would not give us an answer, he would not give a direct answer.

Now, here we are with the "best doctor" in New York for oncology at the best hospital in New York and she is not getting better. Should we try a different approach? No, he tells us, should we stick with the same drugs that don't seem to be working? "Yes", he tells us. Does he explain exactly what is happening? No. Does he tell why now she is getting pain in her bone and her back? No. Not related he says.

As a point of note, I will try and describe what she went through or at least what I saw her go through. In addition to the cancer coming back now two and three times, going through all that chemo, losing her hair twice, all that radiation, being unable to move her left arm because of a biopsy that apparently hit a nerve in the arm, and now 30 pounds lighter, frail looking (although still beautiful). You could see the wear and the difficulty stamped on her face. She was now taking morphine and Oxycontin to try and deaden the pain. She was not getting better. She couldn't eat. She was constipated because of all the drugs they were putting into her system and I can tell you she couldn't go to the bathroom sometimes. Her life was miserable. It was miserable but she was fighting. She wanted to live. We all want to live but we want to live a decent life. We want to live pain free. We want to live with hope. She did too and I wanted that for her more than anything in the world. More than anything in the world.

CHAPTER 6: SLOAN?

Before Mi Song was seen at Columbia Presbyterian and Dr. Oster, she had gone to Sloan Kettering Hospital in New York City to have the cancer removed surgically. This was recommended by doctors at Robert Wood Johnson Hospital and she went over and was to have her cancer removed by a Dr. Bergen who apparently was chief of oncology at the hospital, at least I believe that was his title. She was engaged at the time, as I mentioned previously to a man whose first name was John. I won't give his last name but he was feckless and unworthy of all that Mi was. They (John and Mi) went over for an interview prior to the operation and they had all of the x-rays with them and they made it clear to the doctor, the doctor who was going to do the operation, [Bergen], that there was a concern by the doctors in New Jersey that the cancer was in a spot under her arm and removing it may cause a disability to the arm. Therefore, there was an additional risk in the operation and that was as I just said, that she would lose some strength and movement in her arm unless the surgeon was extremely careful and was able to remove the cancer without interfering with the arm movement.

The operation took place early on a September morning. She went to the hospital quite early with her fiancé [John]. I took a bus from Springfield and went into Port Authority and then took a cab and got up to Sloan about 7:30 in the morning. I was ushered into a small room on the 9th Floor and I was told to wait there and finally they allowed her to come in. She was dressed in a surgical gown and she had not seen me for some time. I gave her a big hug, I wished her good luck and as I was doing that, the nurse is looking rather perplexed. I didn't quite understand why, but she was concerned about the fiancé in the next room. I didn't know he was there, but it didn't matter. The three of us got together to talk about the operation. I gave her a kiss and he and I left and went downstairs to a waiting area. We were told that the operation would last about an hour or an hour and a half and we would be informed when it had been finished and we could come up. Well, we waited. I wasn't especially worried about the operation itself. I was worried primarily that the doctor would get all of the cancer out of there and if he was able to do that, perhaps her life expectancy would be greatly improved. We got a call.

The operation was finished and as we went up to the floor where the operation occurred, to the waiting room, Dr. Bergen came to greet us. I was somewhat concerned as soon as I saw him. I was concerned because it was unusual that the doctor immediately comes out to see you and hands you the x-rays and a pad and pencil. He explained to us that he could not remove all of the cancer. That, he felt that the cancer that was up toward the nerves in the shoulder, he didn't want to take out because it would eventually paralyze that left arm (which did later occur). He put what he called markers on the cancer spot so that when radiation was to begin some weeks later, the person doing the radiation treatment could see more clearly exactly where the cancer was and therefore focus the radiation device more carefully and "kill the cancer!"

CHAPTER 7: FAILURE

Now, although we had concerns about this, I never articulated those concerns to Dr. Bergen. It seems to me and if I look back upon it, it seems to me that the fact that Dr. Bergen, knew, (and he must have known because he saw the x-rays before the operation), if he knew that there was a risk to the shoulder, why didn't he have with him as part of his operating team a neurosurgeon who could have gone in and taken out that cancer and not damage the shoulder. I thought that the fact he did not do that was an indication that he was negligent in the treatment of Mi Song.

Her fiancé and I as soon as we could, went into her room where she was recuperating from the operation. She had not been told that all of the cancer was not taken away. We told her that but put a spin on it. We told her that there was some cancer left and there was a marker on it and that they could eliminate it by using radiation. She seemed happy to hear that and I left the hospital that night after spending another three or four hours with her until they chased me out. I left worrying about that cancer that still remained in and around her shoulder. Little did I know that that was in fact the cancer that would eventually spread and take her life.

When I would go and visit Mi Song at her home as she "recovered" and I tried to do it every day, I went with a good friend of mine, Elaine who would drive me there. She would spend the day there also. We would get to her house early in the morning, maybe about 9:00 a.m. and there was a big sign outside that said WELCOME. I would hunch down as if I was some kind of a large monkey and I would try to chase her around the house. She was frail now, about 30 pounds less than she was a few months before, and she wasn't feeling well, wasn't eating well or sleeping well. Nonetheless, she was able to laugh, run around trying to avoid the "monkey" and we had a good time doing it. I could make her laugh

On the last 'Valentine's Day' of her life, I sent her a card and on the outside of the card, I inscribed the words "My Lion in Winter". In the card I also wrote a short poem to her. She called me and asked, what did that mean? What did the poem mean? Actually, I told her that it really had no meaning. I didn't want to tell her the reason for the poem. The poem really expressed what I felt about what was happening. The poem read as follows:

She walked now over a bridge, broken with age.
As she did, she looked tearfully into a dark sky.
A soft wet snow began to fall on her black hair.
Did I not deal with angels when her tears I touched?
When I kissed her smile?

CHAPTER 8: HER CONVERSION

I even baptized her. One morning at her home she mentioned she would like to be a Christian. I noted that on the table stood a large water glass completely full. "Here is your first day as a Christian", I announced as I placed two fingers into the water in her glass ready to Baptize her. "Come closer and ask Jesus to take your life in His hands." As she did, I placed my moist fingers on her forehead and made the sign of a cross. "You are now a Christian", I said as she looked at me with surprise and some doubt. I was elated.

Chapter 9: Fatal Error

We (Mi and I) had a secret agreement, unknown to her husband. We agreed that if she was going to a hospital or she was going to see a doctor or someone was putting pressure on her to do something that involved an examination of her medical condition, that she would first call me and let me know. I could put my two cents into the picture. She valued my judgment and she knew, absolutely knew that I was faithful to her.

Anyway, I had been down to her home for about seven days at one period in April 2004. I was trying to get her to walk, to have a little more confidence in herself, to build up her strength and to eat more. I left to go home thinking that I was going to take a couple days at my own place and see what was happening there and perhaps come back and stay with her a few days later. I had promised her and her brother's wife who was staying with her, that I would take them to the movies. Mi had not been to the movies in quite a long time.

CHAPTER 10: THREE WEEKS TO LIVE

The following Sunday I was listening to the radio and I heard my phone ring but no one was on the phone. I didn't think anything of it and I went to sleep. The next day I received a phone call from her husband, Marvin. Apparently the night before he took her to a local hospital. Now this not her treating hospital. She was being treated at Columbia Presbyterian. He takes her to a local hospital because she is having a little trouble breathing and I find out that the call that I heard the night before was his call. She had asked him to call me and get in touch with me. He didn't do it. He let the phone ring once and never spoke with me. Now this was what she and I wanted to prevent – i.e., her not getting my input before seeing a new doctor.

Well, he takes her into the hospital and two doctors who had never seen her before, who didn't know her condition, examined her. They took some x-rays apparently and somehow drew fluid out of her lungs through her back. Then they tell her she has three weeks to live! Well, when I heard him tell me that, I almost went insane. I can't describe how I felt. I knew that this was the wrong thing to have done to her. I do not believe that anyone has the right to tell you how long you have to live. That's why I object to much of what goes on in the hospice experience and any doctor who is inclined to do that kind of a thing, I would have nothing to do with him. God decides how long you are going to live. Not some doctor who has had four years of medical school and for all we know, is a C or D student and just about graduated.

I was furious, really, I was furious. I remember going to the hospital where she was the following day and walking into her room. Her sister was with her. Her husband was not there, thank God because I would have strangled that guy. I remember the two of us holding onto each other and crying. I thought to myself, in one day we could have lost, or maybe we have lost everything we worked for. She believed that she was only going to live three weeks. There was nothing I could tell her that would dissuade her. This was the worst thing that could happen to us in terms of attempting to manage her treatment. You don't tell the patient they have three weeks to live. Don't give the patient bad news. You don't have to give them bad news. You can be truthful and spin the news in a way that is acceptable to the patient. You are talking to a victim, you are not talking to some rational individual who can listen, understand and process and grasp for hope. You are talking to someone who is down, someone who has a foot on their throat. They are dying. In other words you are gentle and loving with her but not here. Some fool doctor told her she had three weeks to live.

I called her doctor in New York and told him what they said and by this time I am completely unhappy with him too based upon the predictions and assurances and lack of communication and everything that occurred. He said try and get her in here. See if you can move her from New Jersey and bring her into Columbia Presbyterian. That we could not do. She was now in a total state of collapse. She was not eating, she had lost her hope to live. Her breathing now became extremely difficult. She needed an oxygen tent. Everything followed the fact that she went into a hospital one Sunday night, walking in, Mi feeling pretty good except for a cough but leaving that hospital thinking of death and believing she is going to die in three weeks. To this day, this is something that really bothers me. If that doctor felt that she had three weeks to live, she should have told her husband who was there. Don't tell her. Let the husband decide, even though he was…I'm going to say something very negative about him…a feckless fool. Let me put it this way, if I was there and they told me, first of all I would have told them they don't know what they are talking about. I would have gotten an opinion from her doctor in New York. They didn't know anything about her and if she had to hear three weeks to live, I should have told it to her and I could have said it differently. I could have given her hope at the same time. When you tell a person they have three weeks to live, there is no hope there. That is terrifying and after all that she had been through, all the struggle, all the medication, all the chemotherapy, all the radiation, it was terrible.

CHAPTER 11: HOSPICE

Before I begin to describe what happened to all of us as it became clear that Mi Song's illness was not going to be reversed and that it would take a miracle for her to be healed. Before I get into that I would like to ask a question and this questions troubles me as it has always troubled me. I have no answer for it and I think it troubles many other people who obviously don't have an answer for it and that questions is, "why does a good God allow such suffering"? Whether it is in an individual in their cancer experience or it's in terms of the nation brought to its knees by atomic weapons or a people's life turned upside down because of natural disasters. I always find it humorous to refer to nature as "Mother Nature". Nature is cruel. Nature is no mothering factor. Nature is unpredictable, cruel, angry, and vengeful. Does not take into account good or bad or evil and good. It punishes good as well as evil.

Getting back to the God question, I don't love God because I am afraid of him, I don't think it's too important to me that God can create mankind and the universe. I guess the word important I shouldn't have used but it's not too meaningful to me. I didn't love my father because I was afraid of him. I was afraid that he would punish me or he would inflict corporal punishment on me if I did something wrong. But that is not the reason I loved my father. I loved my father, albeit I knew him only a short time. I loved my dad because he was kind. Because he was forgiving; because he was nurturing and took care of me. Moreover, because I know he cared about my welfare. He tried to send me to the best schools and provide for me and he was loving to my mother and that was significant to me. Now, that is what I look for in God. I want a God who is loving, who is caring, a God who forgives, and a God who although he may have a plan, he does want us to understand that it is a plan that is generally suited for us in terms of our welfare. I don't want a God that I am afraid of. I don't want a God that I am afraid to criticize. I don't want a God that I can't complain to.

I was talking to a cancer patient the other day and she was in her third bout with cancer. She had to have both breasts removed at a fairly young age and I said to her, do you complain to God about this? She kind of laughed and said, oh no. I wouldn't complain or criticize God. I said in response that I would. I said I often say to God, why are you doing something like this? It doesn't make sense. You are supposed to be loving. Why are you destroying people? Why do you take someone's life who cares about you? Why don't you destroy the bad people? We know who they are. You the reader and I know who they are. They are all around us. But they live lives that are happy, at least some of them. They are affluent, healthy. Why is that? I don't have an answer for that. I really don't. I think all we can do is pray for hope and faith. Faith is a gift. You either have it or you don't. I have sometimes little faith. Sometimes I believe there is no God. I believe that you die and that's the end of you. I will never see my mother, my wife or my best friend. I sometimes believe that. I sometimes think of taking my own life.

Think about it for a moment. Jesus took his life. Jesus committed suicide. You say, how is that possible? On the cross Jesus had the ability to save himself. He decided not to. He opted for death. That is what a suicidal person does. They opt for death. They have the ability to save themselves but they kill themselves. So this is the most perplexing problem that I have in my lifetime and I think you probably have in your lifetime. Who is God? What is the meaning of God? Why does God act so capriciously? Why does he act in a way that seems to be contrary to everything we know and love about him?

Again, I have to go back to the fact that we need more faith. God must give us the faith, the strength to go through things that you can't make sense out of and you're angry about it. As I write this book about Mi Song, I get angry. I get angry because she was a beautiful young woman. She was intelligent. She loved God. She was kind. She cared about people and she died. Not only died, but a miserable death as I described previously, a death equal to the pain and suffering Jesus had, maybe worse. Why is that? Many people are going through this. There are 30,000 children dying every day because of hunger or disease. Imagine, it 30,000. What do we care about?

What Hollywood star had a baby yesterday? I am telling you, the human race is defective. We are defective. God made us defective. Why? He built a truck that doesn't run the right way. I don't want to be defective. I want to love everyone. I want everyone to have food, I want everyone to have shelter and be free of pain. Not just the lucky few. We are always in a war. We are always ready to kill people. Look at Iraq. We destroyed that country. They were better off before we got there. Yes, Saddam Hussein was an evil man but we have many evil men in this country. We have war criminals who are idolized in this country. Condoleeza Rice the other day gave a speech welcomed by many yet she's a war criminal. Hundreds of thousands of women and children and old people died in Iraq because of decisions she was making. Her and Bush did that and they look to the bible for their inspiration. Bush reads the bible every morning and prays to God about this. Is there a God anywhere who is agreeing with this? If there is, I tell you now I don't want this kind of God in my life. Bush is misreading what God wants. He has to be. Either he is right or I'm right. Abraham Lincoln in the middle of the Civil War was once approached by a minister from the South. Occasionally Lincoln would allow a Southern officer or preacher to come into the North with a military pass and the minister said to Lincoln, we pray every morning for our success. Lincoln looked at him and paused for a moment and said, "we pray every morning for our success." Lincoln looked at him again and said, "somebody is praying to the wrong God". Think of that for a moment, the South thought that they were righteous, that slavery was an institution supported by the bible. In their churches they were being told that was correct. When they prayed to God, they believed that it was a correct position for them to take. It wasn't. God blessed the North. God wanted union, he didn't want slavery. Think about these things. There may come a day when, if Jesus is to be believed. He will come again and instill upon the earth a government that is fair and just. All people will live in peace and harmony. All people will have food and water. All people will have access to education. Either that or he will destroy us all and create something good. The earth is not a good place. There is no Mother Nature. There is no absence of evil. There is no absence of war. There is evil all around us. There is evil inside of us. Each of us has the ability to commit any crime that ever was committed. That's what the Lord's Prayer means by, "lead us not into temptation". Christ is saying pray to God that you may avoid evil.

CHAPTER 12: PRAYER

"Oh death has come with only its rain and ruin, flowers are slain and frosts begotten. She is gone and I know not where."

I would like to comment about the meaning of prayer, especially when one is going through circumstances that are really testing your belief. When I was young, especially when I went into grade school, I went to a Catholic school taught by the sisters and I basically learned two prayers. The first was the Our Father and the second was the Hail May and for much of my life I used those two prayers in an attempt to reach God or to at least get God to pay attention to what I needed or as a way of simply adoring God. As I am older, I of course realize there are many ways to pray. As I talk to people who respond to my TV or radio programs and they tell me that they find it hard to pray. I suggest to them that perhaps much of what they do during the day is in fact, a prayer. For example, you can pray by complaining.

Doesn't that seem strange that I am saying to you that you can go and complain to God and that is a prayer? Indeed it is. Picture yourself as a parent for example and one of your children comes to you and complains that they have just fallen down and are bleeding. That's a complaint. You listen to that, you try and heal that and do all you can for that child. You may have a child who comes and complains about a sibling. You will do something about that. You will try to again to give kind words to that child. God is really the same way, I think. A million times more accepting. God understands that you are human. God understands that you feel pain. God understands that tragedy is really interfering with and sometimes destroying your life. You have a right to say to God, why me? Why do I get all of these problems and I see the woman across the street and nothing seems to go wrong for her. I live a Christian life. I go to church and I pray you tell God. I try and treat my neighbors fairly. I reach out if I can. Why me? I think that's a legitimate prayer and I also think that it's a legitimate prayer even if you are not suffering any particular problem other than listening to what's going on in the world. The thing that always amuses me is you will hear of an earthquake or a tidal wave that will kill thousands of people and someone on the television, will say, well Mother Nature, get this, Mother Nature has done something again.

What is this Mother Nature myth? Nature is not a mother. Nature is cruel. Nature is capricious. Nature is not God. God creates all of the factors that lead to a hurricane perhaps and he did that billions of years ago but God doesn't cause the hurricane. God is not destroying nations with earthquakes. I would ask you the question, "tell me when God prayed?"

Think about this for a minute. When, for example did Jesus pray and if he did, do you know what words he used? I can tell you that you don't know. When Jesus went into the desert for thirty days of fasting and prayer, we don't know what he said. The bible doesn't tell us. Indeed, Jesus recommends that we learn and pray the Our Father but he didn't pray the Our Father at that particular time with his disciples. It was a recommendation. Only the words were told to them.

So, you tell me now, when did Jesus pray. I want to know what words did Jesus use that are stated in the bible that were words of prayer. Was it the Hail Mary? No. Was it the Our Father? No. I am going to give you one example of where I know Jesus prayed. Jesus was in the Garden of Gethsemane about to be taken away and tortured With his death looming, a painful and horrible death, Jesus prayed, and we know that

Jesus said to the Father, "if You can remove this cup from my lips, please remove this". Just think of that kind of a prayer. That is the kind of prayer you can use every day. You talk to Jesus as if he is a person. You don't walk up to a priest and kneel down and start saying the Hail Mary, and you don't have to do it with Jesus either. The Our Father, of course, is a beautiful prayer, but you don't have to talk to God that way.

So there is an example of God praying, and I will give you one more. Just before He died on the cross, He looked to the heavens and He asked God to take His spirit, to finally take His life. It was over. Do it now. Take it, I've had enough. Why can't we talk to God like that? If you are reading this and you know you have cancer or someone in your family has cancer or someone is ill from some other disease, ask God to take it away. Take it away. That's how we pray. We are human.

I many times in my life get angry with God. Many times I question this Mother Nature nonsense. Many times I ask why 30,000 children die of hunger and other disease every day. Why? Why does a good God allow that? Then I ask God to do something about it. Stop it. Take it away. Give them relief. We can't go on like this. I wish He would come, I do, and I really do. Get rid of this dystopia that's here.

CHAPTER 13: MI'S PROPHECY

I had a serious relationship with Mi Song, and as a result of that, we became very good friends and I think I have stated earlier that we had planned to marry at one point. She would tell me that she had experiences as a young girl seeing things and understanding things that would become apparently true later on in her lifetime. Her father was deceased at an early age due to cancer and she told me that there was a garden in the back of her home in Korea and she would visit the garden at night and she would see her father there and her father would appear to her. Her father would talk to her about perhaps family problems or solutions that she needed to hear.

Much more significant to me however, was what she told me, as she went into the cancer experience. She guaranteed to me that she knew, and I assumed she was telling me through some type of revelation, (a spiritual and supernatural revelation) that she was not going to die of the cancer. Now, of course she did die of the cancer and as I think about it today, that does not reflect negatively on her prophetic feeling about that, because there are a number of ways to die. In my opinion, she never completely died. In my opinion she is living here with me as I dictate this memory. I feel her presence often. I know she is not dead. She is perhaps in a different dimension. She is somewhere that I can't reach as a human. Hopefully this is a place I will be able to reach when I die.

I was thinking this morning of a simple prayer that Jesus told us to use when praying when he was asked. How do we pray? He told us how by introducing to the human race forever the concept of the Our Father as a prayer. There are many ways to understand the Our Father and I am going to take a few minutes now to go through it. Mi Song interpreted the Our Father for me. Now I had knowledge of the Our Father for half a century and she was not a Christian and she had only come upon it fairly recently. Yet her insights were much more powerful and meaningful than mine and I am going to share them with you. The opening line is "Our Father who art in heaven". Now the concept of father (Jesus using that as a metaphor for the ruler of the universe) as opposed to a mother, or as opposed to nature, or as opposed to Jesus himself. Father as used by Jesus is a concept that means both love, respect, punishment when called for, but just punishment, no cruelty, and empathy. It invokes in us and it is meant to invoke in us, the belief that we have an approachable God. A God whom we can go to with all of our misery, our failings, our anger, our joy whatever it happens to be. And as a father, our God will accept us. Now that is a wonderful thing because it means that some of the thinking that is part of the fundamentalist interpretation of the bible, namely that we have a harsh, punishing God and you must fear God is error. I know that when I was in Catholic grammar school, the Nuns taught us that you have to be afraid of God. God was watching you all the time and if you did anything wrong, you were going to be punished. Frankly, it was God that I was fearful of and this is not what Jesus is telling us. Jesus is telling us that we have a loving, caring, accepting, flexible Father and that we should go to the Father. He is our Father. Think about your own childhood and your own father and believe that he is someone you can talk to. Hopefully he is someone who is willing to listen, forgive, offer solutions to help you and that's really what Jesus was telling us about God the Father.

"Hallowed be Thy name" –now what is Jesus saying there? I said to Mi Song, "what is Jesus trying to tell us here?" The word hallowed means, of course, that you place the name of God the Father in a very special category. Then I said to her, "why is it a special category? You just got done telling me that God the Father is to be seen as my father was, loving and caring. Her answer was that the difference is that you don't question what God the father tells you and you don't blaspheme against Him just because things are going wrong in your life. Many times I was upset with my own father. To this day, I believe there are certain decisions that he made that were wrong and that his personality could have been improved. These are feelings that we may have about our God in heaven but we are supposed to re-examine that and believe that it's not true, that there is no defect in this God. Unlike our father, his name should be Hallowed in the sense that he has no defects. Every father who is human has a defect. Not the least of which is the original sin that apparently, at least according to Biblical teaching has created all of the woes in the world, including the need that we have to die and often die in pain.

"Thy Kingdom Come"—is nothing that I recall her making too much of a comment about except that God will cleanse the earth at some time. That God will place his own sense of justice and rule and fairness upon the earth. I welcome that and look forward to it. God will end the conflict, end the wars..."thy Kingdom come, thy will be done". God's will is always done.

One of the things we talk about in discussions with cancer patients or in our own foundation and philosophies is the fact that it is not the doctor or the nurse who decides whether you are going to live or die. Mi Song was told she had three weeks to live by a doctor and I have discussed earlier how disastrous this was in terms of her own psychology. He had no right to say how long she had to live. "Thy Will Be Done." God will decide, not a doctor.

Perhaps a prayer could change God's mind. Think of that. Why else do you pray? You pray really saying to God most of the time, there is something wrong in my life and I am having trouble with it can you fix it? Can you change it or do something about it? Of course, He can. But we are also realistic and God's will may not be your will. God's will may not be what you are feeling. God's will may be that you are going to suffer a death. Why would God allow you to die and suffer. God has his motives and the Jesuits used to tell me that God writes in crooked lines. We don't know.

"Lead us not into temptation." What does that mean? That simply means that you seek to be insulated from temptation or opportunity to do wrong. Even the best among us if tempted vigorously will sin. Only Jesus (and he was tempted by Satan) could resist and remain sin free. It means that when you pray to God, you ask to not experience things that put you to the test. For example, assume that you were a Nazi soldier in World War II and you are fighting in a battlefield situation. Assume also you have been told since you have been a child that the Jewish race is a race that has to be watched carefully and if necessary, segregated. In fact, the Catholic church itself took the position (until recently) that the Jews were responsible for the death of Christ. Martin Luther, the founder of the Protestant movement and a Catholic priest took the position that God hated Jews and that the Jews could not go to heaven. Assume you grew up in a country believing this and Germany was a Protestant, Lutheran/Catholic country. Suppose your family believed that. So here, you are, you are ordered to execute a Jewish prisoner and you do.

As you hear me relate this story to you, do you say you could not possibly do something like that? God is saying to you, pray to me so you are not placed in that kind of situation—so you don't have to make a judgment about this kind of thing. I do not believe that people who do things that objectively can be characterized as evil are evil. I do not believe that these people are necessarily evil. My son once said to me, let me put it to you this way, let's assume that we have a race and the prize is $1 million, just the two of us. It's a hundred yard race. The only exception is that you can only race with one leg. Who is going to win that race? When you lose that race can you be criticized for that? Can you be punished by losing the $1 million? I would suggest to you that "do not lead us into temptation" means don't put me in a race with only one leg.

Chapter 14: Death

Death is probably one of the most difficult things that you can talk to a cancer victim about. I tried to avoid it as much as I could when I was with Mi Song, especially in the early years of her cancer. Much to my surprise however, she seemed to be quite willing to discuss death. Finally, we both agreed that we would talk about it and I was especially interested to receive her view on this. I am not sure how I feel about it. Some days I don't want to die. Some days I wish I was not living. I surely don't wish to die in pain. I don't wish to suffer and frankly if it came down to that, if I had the choice of suffering or dying, I would die. I would take my own life if I thought that it would avoid suffering. She did not feel that way. She, in her long struggle with cancer, which had lasted over three years, only at one point did she indicate that she wanted to kill herself. That was when she was being treated by a physician with acupuncture and manipulation as opposed to painkillers. The pain in her shoulder where the cancer was living and killing her was so great that she had suicidal thinking at that time. That was the only time.

I remember about two weeks before she died, we were sitting on the couch in her living room and she said to me, "I accept my death". That was a statement I can tell you that astonished me. I didn't know what to say to her. I would always say to her when I had the opportunity and I wasn't caught by surprise, I would always say the words, "you are not going to die". We are going to keep you alive. There are plenty of alternatives, there are new medicines. There are new medicines being tested, experimental and we will try anything we can. I will take you to anywhere, you are simply not going to die. Most of the time she accepted that. But as she got more morphine addicted, as a result of her pain, I think she began to take a different view as to whether or not her life meant that much to her anymore. We discussed what happens to you after you died. We both agreed that you didn't feel anything, the heart stopped and as a result all of the nerve endings in your body would die and there would be no pain sensation anywhere. You would eventually over a period of years, end up as dust or nothing at all.

But, we also believed that there was another dimension surrounding us and that people who had died before us, people who were meaningful to us were there somewhere and that we would all meet up in that dimension. A nice, fanciful idea of dying. I would love to think about that. I'm not sure if it's true or I believe it but she felt that it was true. She felt that she was able to tap into that dimension from time to time. The problem that I had with her dying, among all the other problems I had with it, was losing a wonderful friend and seeing her die in so much pain. The fear I had with seeing anyone dying was that that soul would be lost forever. I have a short poem in my mission statement that simply says that "only she was she", which is true. There will never be another Mi Song. God would never create another and the one who existed and the one I knew is now gone forever. That is what really burdens me for the rest of my life.

Timothy Leary, I think he was a PhD, from Harvard, the founder of the LSD movement in the 60's and who died about ten years ago, was looking forward to his death. He anxiously awaited his death because he knew he was going to pass into a new existence and he felt that was going to be quite exciting. Montaigne called it on his deathbed, "la Grand Peut-etre", (the great unknown) which was about to happen. Nietzsche, the German philosopher felt that sometimes death was preferable to life and in fact, the willingness that a person might have to kill themselves was a way to get through some of the most horrific things in your life because nothing could be so difficult that you couldn't deal with it by killing yourself. Socrates, just before committing suicide was asked, "what is going to happen to you?" He said there are only two possibilities and I am happy with both of them. One is that I don't exist anymore and I will have no feeling and I won't know about it. The other is that there is another dimension and I will go there and live happily in that dimension.

This indirectly takes us to the hospice experience. In Hospice, generally the doctor places you there or decides you should be in the experience and now is willing to staff it with nurses who really sit on a death watch over you. Generally he is putting you into a morphine situation. They increase the drug level, eliminating your pain and eventually you die. We object to the hospice situation because we feel that it should not be a death watch, but a life watch. We think that everything should be done in the hospice experience to keep you alive and to keep hope strong as opposed to saying, well, this is the end of the road and this is the last stop before the patient dies. We don't believe in that. We believe that God decides when you will die. We believe that no matter how sick you might be that you can still turn it around and get healthy. There are hundreds and hundreds of examples of people who were on their death bed, their last breath and yet they became healthy again. So, I like to be optimistic about that and I am optimistic only because I believe that God runs everything and God will decide life or death.

Finally, if there is a God and I have made it clear that I believe there is and Mi Song believed that there was. If there is a God, after you die you will be treated fairly. You are going to be treated as your dad, your father would treat you if after your death you came to him for a decision as to what the rest of your existence would be like. We must believe in God. It's not only good for us spiritually but good for us psychologically. No one has ever been able to prove that there is no God. You can argue until you are blue in the face and you still cannot prove that. Believing in God and knowing that the greatest gift you can receive (and this is what you should pray for) is the gift of faith. And it is the ability to believe that there is a God and that God is interested in you is the greatest gift of all. Faith. Pray for that.

CHAPTER 15: FINAL THOUGHTS
A VISIT WITH MI

I dictate this on a Sunday, the 16th of September 2012 and I visited the gravesite of Mi Song today. I had not been there and it's hard for me to explain why, for almost five years. It is also her birthday today and that's primarily the reason I went on this day. This day too marked another anniversary, not a birthday but a death day, the death of my brother, 58 years ago today. He was sixteen. What I always found remarkable about this day, was that I know Mi Song was born on this day and my brother, as I mentioned died on this day. In fact, it happened almost at the very same time. The time my brother died, Mi Song was being born. I didn't really think about that very much until after she had died. It was a signal to me that there was a connection here and that connection although it was not conscious on my part, that connection drew me closer to Mi Song.

My son Joseph came with me and we traveled together to the grave. It was a beautiful day. It was sunny with a light wind. It's not cold. The sky was beautiful with very few clouds. It's early September. As I recall back when Mi Song died, (she died in May) the days are almost the same as I remember. Going to a cemetery for me is always difficult. My wife was now buried in a cemetery close by me and in fact, I go there as often as I can. I am not driving and I do find it difficult to go but I just feel there is something I should be able to say, something I should be able to do to draw them out

of the ground and bring them back to life. I feel
angry when I go the cemetery. Sometimes I feel
angry because God took these two people at such a
young age. Mi Song was not fifty years old when
she had to die a terrible death.

There is anger in me. I touched the stone, as I
always do, (and the heavy granular feeling that one
gets when they touch a grave stone) it creates a
new sadness. I remove my hand quite quickly
because of that. I look at the dates on the stone
and I put my cross there as I did today into Mi
Song's gravesite. I have a cross that I had on her
grave when she died that I took back for a while
just so I could keep a piece of her but I put it back
again today and I will take it back again in a year
or two. My rancor soon turns to sadness. I sit
down next to the grave and remember what kind of
person she was and how life can be so difficult for
some people and yet today I don't come to any
conclusions about it. I just sit there and wonder,
question and remember. But you don't conclude
anything; there is no finality to it. You'll be back
again, the memories will come back. The sadness
will come back. The anger will always be there.
The day I die and I come before God, if that
happens, he will know there is still anger in me.

My brother died young too. I remember that
night. I was seventeen years old and he was going
on sixteen. We were very close and I remember
kneeling outside of my home after he died. It was
dark and there was a full moon. Looking at the
moon I hoped that someone (I didn't know why he
died at that time) but I hoped someone perhaps
took his life with their car. I would be able to find

that person and I would be able to bring my own justice upon that person. That would make me feel okay. Then I would have paid my brother back. I didn't care what God had to say about it. I wasn't interested in God's justice, I was interested in my justice.

It was the same thing when Mi Song died. It's not incorrect to say that I visited the cemetery once a week for two years, religiously. I came before they had the stone there, I had something made up for her so I would know who was in the grave. The ring that my mother took from my father's finger when he died, the ring that she gave him on their engagement, the ring I wore for so many years, I buried with Mi Song. I was angry then too. I was angry at the doctor, I was angry at the hospital, I was angry at the treatment she received. I was angry at her husband.

If I had, and thank God I didn't, if I had the means to take my anger out on someone, perhaps I would have done that. But I didn't. I suffered with it, I still suffer. I am angry as I dictate this. The anger and disappointment that I have with the medical profession, with doctors who don't care about people but care about what you can pay, what your insurance card looks like. They care about a steak they are going to have for dinner that night. They didn't think about Mi Song. Very few people loved Mi Song. I loved Mi Song. It wasn't a carnal love, rather it's talked about in the Christian churches as "agape". It was the kind of love that God has for us. I loved Mi Song. I hate these days. But there is something in this day that tells me that they are safe. God loves her too. He is protecting. If only that would give me support and the ability to sleep at night. Not always.

I left her grave and promised her that I would go back again and I will go back. She can still count on me. That was the bond that existed between us. I will be back and after my death will be there with her.

Chapter 16: After Mi's Death

Before her funeral, I gave a small talk at the wake that was difficult for me to do. I was in so much disbelief and shock yet I still decided to say a few words. Anyone who has tried to do that kind of thing, realizes how impractical it is. You cannot summarize in a few sentences, in a few minutes, in a few hours, everything that you feel and have felt, and have known about that person. In addition to an emotional feeling, you cannot get through the eulogy without showing your emotions.

I do recall that her body was behind us. She was in a red dress and looked so beautiful as I walked over and touched her hand. I regret to this day that I did not kiss her, but I didn't. Her family was sitting up in front and when I began to express my feelings, I heard her brother sob which was unusual for him. He was a strong young Korean man who fought in the Korean army. It was something that was not expected. I got through it and the ceremony ended and we proceeded to take her body to the cemetery.

I helped carry the casket. The one thing I noticed was that it was extremely heavy. That surprised me. There were four men, four of us carrying the casket and yet for me it seemed extremely heavy. Probably symbolic of the fact that I was carrying to the grave someone who was that important to me. I recall vaguely now being at the cemetery. I watched them lower her body into the grave. I think if it wasn't for the Xanax I had, I could not have kept my composure. Although her family members were Buddhists and although we did not have a Christian burial, I said out loud the Our Father in front of the grave and the people who were there who were familiar with the prayer, joined in.

CHAPTER 17: KILLING

Much about what happened is much clearer today than it was back then. I am writing this, in part to warn the reader of the pitfalls that exist in cancer treatment. In fact, this is true for any treatment in hospitals by doctors in this country and I suspect in any country. For examples, I did not know at that time that at least 100,000 people lose their lives every year as a result of the negligence of either a doctor or nurse in the hospital setting. That means you can go into the hospital with an ailment, and it might have been a minor ailment yet you die from something that they do wrong in the hospital. Not only do they cover this up, but it is very difficult to get this information. As I dictate this, President Obama has passed new Health Care legislation. This will force hospitals to disclose this kind of negligence and if they don't, they will lose part of their Medicare reimbursement.

Now, the same thing is true for the physicians. A patient who is being treated for cancer, (and I am going to stay on the cancer issue, because that is the issue that concerns me) a patient who is being treated for cancer does not know whether or not that doctor who is treating him or her has past litigation against him for negligence. They don't know what his qualifications are. They don't know whether his practice has been suspended in certain hospitals. They should know this! Again, that information is not readily available. My foundation, the Mi Song Memorial Cancer Foundation gathers all of this information into a computer data base so that if a patient comes to us and that patient tells us what hospital they are being treated at, what doctor is treating them and what drug is being used, we can research all of that and we can give them some important information that may in fact, suggest to them that they go somewhere else, have a different doctor or go to a different hospital.

Do you know, for example, that doctors are often paid by drug companies, a kickback or a bonus if that doctor will prescribe the drug that is being manufactured by that particular drug company? For example, let's say you have cancer and let's say your doctor is using drug A on you to treat that cancer. Now there is a possibility (and if that possibility exists, you should know about it) there is a possibility that that doctor has at his disposal, other drugs that he is not using because he is not getting kickbacks on those drugs. He is getting a kickback on the drug that he is using, a drug that is being recommended by the drug company and their salesperson, the outside representative who comes to his office and sells that drug to him. What we are saying is that we want you to be in the best possible situation, we want you to have the best doctor and we want you to be using the best modality, the best drug, yet there may be no way that you can make sure you are doing this.

Finally, we have listed in the appendix to this book, sources found both on the internet and other places that you can go to on your own to try and determine whether not the doctor you are using or the hospital that you are in is of the qualify that you feel is necessary to your care. For example, U.S. News and World Report indicate that the top four hospitals are in the New York area as well as some of the worst hospitals. That report indicates that the worst hospital is Jacoby and the top hospital is Columbia Presbyterian. You should know these things. There is also a publication in New York called New York Magazine and every year they rank the 100 best doctors in the tri-state area. Now be careful with that, this is an internal ranking. Doctors rank each other and may not be objective. For example, when Mi Song was being treated at Columbia Presbyterian, we used a Dr. Oster who apparently was nominated by New York Magazine ten years in a row for oncology. In fact, we found him to be quite poor and was the object of litigation, by us, as a result of that. So you have to be careful, you have to do your own research.

If you can't do that, you can come to us. The Mi Song Cancer Foundation. You can find us on the web, www.misongfoundation.org. You can Google Professor Joseph Masterson and you can find us on Christian radio and television. You can also find us on family radio and on YouTube. If you do your research, you can help yourself very much.

This book is, in my opinion, an indictment against the medical profession and the pharmaceutical industry. They are not doing the best possible job that can be done. The war on cancer was begun under the Nixon administration and still continues. There hasn't been much progress. People are dying of cancer just as much today as they ever were, perhaps even more so.

There is not much that we have learned and it is going to continue. It will continue as long as the drug companies are profit motive driven and as long as the doctors are willing to collaborate with the drug companies and not do what is best for you, it will continue as long as we have poor quality hospitals. Everything has to be cleaned up. If it isn't we are going to see death rates from cancer that go on and on. Remember the statistics I gave you before. One hundred thousand people die in hospitals from the negligence of nurses and doctors. Many hospitals themselves are unclean. When we took Mi Song to Columbia Presbyterian, it took us three years to find out that at the very time she was being treated there, there was Legionnaire's Disease in the hospital water supply and they were keeping it quiet. Imagine that!

CHAPTER 18: HER POETRY

When I first met "Mugga" I wrote some poetry and as I looked through my notes, I came across a piece that I think describes the way I felt about her during our initial meeting and also for a brief time after that when I in fact, learned that she had cancer. Seeing how much she had struggled, I wrote:

> "Three tear soaked sacks filled with
> heavy black iron were placed upon a
> tiny back as all the cares under
> heaven fell upon her."

The cancer had not taken away from her the beauty that she possessed. It is obvious that when one saw her that she was one of the most beautiful woman you had ever seen. At least that was true for me and I wrote one evening after spending a few hours with her,

> "And God sent an Asian rose petal with
> but gentle thorns, as sweet as the
> Eastern air could make her was she."

In addition, I wrote,

> "This garden is ever so fresh now made
> fragrant too all because my darling
> sleeps here".

I believe that was the quote I wrote after she had died and probably is not congruent with the previous quotes, but I will keep it there.

Another I wrote was:

> "Spring and its gardens were in her
> every smile. She had black evening hair
> but a bright morning heart. Her lips

were cherry red, a voice of silk and
honey."

This was the impression that you would get
when you saw her. Indeed this was true
throughout the cancer experience. I remember one
day when I was with her she was visited by a friend
she had known for many years, about her same
age. The friend of course was more energetic,
bouncing back and forth in her living room, and Mi
whispered to me, "I wish I could look pretty like
that". I looked at her and I said to her, "you are
much prettier than she is". "She has spent hours
putting on makeup and fixing her hair, you haven't
done that." Mi always remained beautiful to me.

As her cancer progressed, my poetry and my
writings became more maudlin, more serious and
sad, for example, here is something I wrote at a
time when she was taking her cancer treatments.

"My poor Korean butterfly, flight for only
a brief time, wings once golden with
kisses of purple and summer green are
now broken, ripped and torn. Lo at this
garden spot rests the ever delight of my
heart, till I see her again, I shall not love
red roses, I will loathe sweet tunes."

Some poetry written about that time was
something that I put on a Valentine's Day card
that I sent to her, and I remember her calling me
and asking me what it meant. I was referring to
her at that time as my "Lion in Winter". It was in
the winter of her life that she was a true lion. She
had the courage of ten men. Nothing could cause
fear in her. She was not afraid to die, I was afraid,
she wasn't. She was the strongest woman I had

ever met in my lifetime. What I wrote to her that Valentine's Day, would be the last Valentine's Day that we would ever share together, I wrote:

"She walked now alone over a bridge broken with age. As she did, she looked fearfully into a dark sky. A soft wet snow began to fall on her

black hair. Did I not deal with angels when her tear I kissed when I touched her smile?"

CHAPTER 19: VISITATION

I have vivid memories. I can almost see myself with her now. I remember two weeks after she had died, I was not sleeping well in those days and I had the feeling that she was at the side of my bed trying to speak to me. I sat up and indeed I saw her. She was all in black and for a long time during our relationship she called me "Nerdy Professor" but never Joseph. She said "I love you very, very much Joseph." Those were her exact words. I touched her hand and my impression was it was cold. I tried to keep her there but she vanished. I have never seen her again. I cried.

After she died I wrote a number of pieces of poetry. I will now state them here:

"Oh death has come with rain and ruin, flowers are slain and frosts begotten. She is gone and I know not where. I whispered to her, if death and grave must meet you, they must take not one but two, now the grave that gave her rest at least beckoned him too but with a lover's smile."

"While the lingering winter chilled the lap of May, cruel nature has at this spot placed my poor darling. She was yet in the fresh blush of her perfection."

"And when she dies we will hold her and kiss her and then break her into a thousand tiny stars and placing them into the darkest night the earth will glow bright forever. There will be no need for a morning sun."

"This garden now, ever so fresh grows violets too made more fragrant all because my darling rests here."

CHAPTER 20: MORE FEELINGS

"We fell out she and I, oh we fell out I know not why, we now kiss again but only in tears, longing so for the touch of vanished hands and the sounds of her voice now so still."

"Pray whistle me a melody stranger," said I as I passed four iron gates shutting out a cold black wind. "No stranger sir am I," came the reply, rather said she "I am the love you search for, come sit with me, I will calm all your fears."

"Is it better Mi not to be? Is this slumber more sweet to you than our toil? Is death welcome that puts an end to your pain. Ah but I do remember you. Shut always within the bosom of the rose. To look at you was to love you and to love you was also to be."

"We both believed what we could not prove, waken therefore thou, come home again, you were my soul, the grace of my day, come back to me. Is your slumber now more sweet to you than our toil? Listen carefully my melancholy heart speaks unto me. Is it better not to be than to be?"

"And so it was that cruel nature placed upon a tiny back three sacks filled with years of the heaviest black iron. She wept as all cares under heaven fell upon her. Did I not deal with angels in knowing her? Do angels tear? Do angels suffer?"

"My tears that punish me now forever and forever. I am looking today on our summer times and thinking of the days that are no more. Days as dear as remembered kisses. Kisses my love that would wake the dead and tempt me out of my gloom. Kisses red and moist, never enough."

"She was in her summer bloom, a sight indeed to craft an old man young again. I often felt that if I could only pluck and hold that dear flower in my hand, root and all, I would truly know what God is. But alas God's finger touched her and she slept."

"This dust was once the girl. She was the only mortal shut within the bosom of the rose. Such a one I do remember whom to look at was also to love and to love her was also to be."

"I was in my chilled age but she was in her summer bloom. She was like the morning glory of a happy winter, a sight indeed to craft an old man young again. If I could pluck and hold that dear flower in my hand, root and all, I would surely know what God was and what men are. But alas, like a fluttered bird she was gone. "Oh sweet is death" she called out to me "who puts an end to my pain". Now God's finger touched hers and she slept."

"She wore in her heart the white flower of a life without blame I try to put into words the grief I feel but words only half reveal my soul within. A soul once nourished by a simple girl now dead while in her flower."

"Do you see this dust? This dust on this small hill was once the girl. In her every aspect she was set with but gentle thorns, as sweet the Eastern air could make her. Ah, she was a girl worth dying for."

"This girl was once my glory let it be remembered I was once owned of thee."

She is sleeping: "At last the trouble and the turmoil is over, she is sleeping at last. The struggle and harrow is now past. She is cold and white. She is out of friends and lovers. Out of sight of both but she is sleeping at last."

At Mia's Grave: "My God what evil thing, what craven act has taken more from me than ever was or ever could be. How I Am Stricken. Where is that sweet voice that made home in my memory past? Would that cruel nature have made only one copy."

Mi at Peace: "She is now awakened from the dream called life. She lives, she wakes, tis death which dies, not she. She is forever now a portion of all she once made whole. She is the morning star which once was bright upon the living but now in death she is the evening star which shines upon the dead. She has been made the bride of nature, there can be heard in her voice all nature's music, from thunderous deep moans to the song of the night's sweet birds."

Mi Song at Rest: "Warm summer sun shine softly here. Warm southern winds blow ever gently. Soil above press light, press light. Goodnight sweet Korea, goodnight. She was as perfect in her bud as in her bloom."

"My poor Korean butterfly. You had flight for only a brief time. Your wings once golden with kisses of purple and summer greens are now broken, ripped and torn. Lo at this garden spot rests the ever delight of my heart, till I see her again I shall not love red roses, I will loathe sweet tunes."

"Oh death has come with only its rain and its ruin. Flowers are slain and frosts begotten. She is gone and I know not where."

"He whispered to her "If death and grave must meet you, they must take not one but two." Now the grave that gave her rest at last, beckoned him too but with a lover's smile."

"While the lingering winter chilled the lap of May, cruel nature has at this spot laid my poor darling. She was yet in the fresh blush of her perfection."

"Spring and its gardens were in her every smile. She had black evening hair but a bright morning heart. Lips of cherry red, a voice of silk and honey had she."

"And when she dies, we will hold her and kiss her and then of her make a thousand tiny stars and placing them into the darkest night, fill the world bright forever. No more need for a morning sun."

"She walked now alone over a bridge broken with age. As she did she looked tearfully into a dark sky. Wet snow began to fall on her black hair. Did I not deal with angels when her tear I touched? When I kissed her smile?"

CHAPTER 21: REDEUX
THOUGHTS ABOUT GOD

There is a God, I believe, or at least I believe there should be one. I also believe that God is good and just. I look at my own life however, and I see so much sadness, pain and tragedy. I ask myself how can a good God do this to me? Have I been so offensive, have I been so wayward that God feels I need to be punished? But then I look at others, I look at Mi Song. I stayed with her for the entire length of her cancer and her death. She suffered much more than I ever suffered. Her faith was stronger. She never doubted that there was a God. She never doubted that God loved her. I look at the world in general. It's a terrible place. People hate people, if you have money and success you are fairly safe. Even then, God punishes people drastically. So, to answer my question, is there a God? Yes, I believe there is a God or there should be a God.

CHAPTER 22:
A BRIEF BIOGRAPHY OF MI SONG
"NEVER ENOUGH"

Mi Song was born in South Korea on September 16, 1964. She was born into a middle class family, a family that had seen hardship and struggle especially when one realizes that the country was occupied by the Japanese for many years prior to enduring the Second World War. In Korea at that time, and probably today, men were valued more than women. It was highly unusual to see a woman scholastically superior and who was physically superior. There were many beautiful women in South Korea and of course Mi Song was beautiful. She was also excellent in school. So excellent in fact that her father remarked to her mother once, "she must be a boy." She excelled in sports, long distance running and sprinting. She participated in the Olympics. She was a national beauty contestant. She in fact even sang on Korean radio.

As life goes, she met a U.S. Army Captain and came to the U.S. and started a life here. She would bring with her some years later, her brother and her sister. The three of them together would participate in this great American experiment which still continues to this day. She could speak four languages when she arrived. She had a college education. She was young and healthy and beautiful. She had everything to look forward to.

As she entered her 40th year, she began to notice that she had hardness in her breasts. It was diagnosed as breast cancer and for the next three or four years she would fight that cancer even though it returned on three separate occasions. I saw her lose 30 pounds and she was only a tiny girl to begin with. I saw her cry often. I saw great lumps on her chest, testimony to the evil cancer that existed in her body. But I saw great courage. She never doubted that she would win the fight with this cancer. We saw many doctors and we were in a number of hospitals and the part of this book that I feel is one of the most important parts is the fact that today I am convinced that doctors and hospitals fail with their patients. Nonetheless, she continued through treatment and after some horrible and painful days, she died on May 27, 2004.

Before she died, she and I discussed creating a foundation, a foundation that would be an informational source to people suffering with cancer. We would try and make sure patients knew who the best doctors and, hospitals were and the best kinds of medicines that they should be taking. That is the mission of the Mi Song cancer foundation which exists today and will exist forever. It is her guiding spirit, her courage, her determination that has made this all possible.

CHAPTER 23: ABOUT THE AUTHOR
"SINE APOLOGIA"

The author, Joseph Masterson was born in Bayonne, New Jersey and is the oldest of five children. He was educated in Catholic Parochial grammar schools, went to a military high school in New York City (Xavier High School) and graduated from Wagner College with a B.A. in Psychology with honors. He attended Brooklyn Law School on a scholarship, was published as a member of the Law Review and was cited by the California Supreme Court (a rare occasion for a law student). He graduated Brooklyn Law School with honors, went to New York University, and received an advanced teaching degree (L.L.M.). After law school, he was counsel to the M.W. Kellogg Co., Hoffman LaRoche, Inc, in New Jersey and was asked by the Dean of his law school to join the faculty. This request by the Dean was made at a time when he was only 27 years old which would have made him one of the youngest Law Professors in the country. He did not join the law school faculty until 1972. When he came to the law school in 1972 he was the first to introduce the course in antitrust law and the antitrust law seminar. He was to teach those courses for the next 22 years, becoming a full professor in 1985.. In addition to teaching, he founded his own business, (Professional Seminar Associates) and he spoke on anti-trust sales and marketing restrictions throughout the United States to senior executives in major corporations. Professional

Seminar Associates existed until 1992. In addition, Professor Masterson was an administrative law judge of the City of New York, as well as a certified federal mediator out of the Eastern District of New York. He too was special counsel appointed by Judge Leo Glasser, sitting at the Federal District Court in the Eastern District. Professor Masterson is also the Chairman and President of the Mi Song Cancer Foundation. He lives in New Jersey and his wife of 40 years who is now deceased has a special place in the foundation. Her name was Mary Masterson. Professor Masterson met Mi Song in the year 1997 when he was giving a lecture on Abraham Lincoln before the Historical Society of Westfield New Jersey and they remained friends until her death and now until forever.

President's Comment

The thoughts and feelings about Mi Song here in poetic prose reflect the special place she had, and continues to have, in the Mission of this Foundation and in my heart and life. You, the reader, have someone too who holds you dear. If you, on the other hand, find yourself alone, accept God into your life and struggle. The Mi Song Foundation is here to help with this too. Only you are you! Don't die! ™

Joseph S. Masterson, B.A., J.D., LL.M.
President and C.E.O. of the Mi Ryung Song Memorial Cancer Foundation
(Professor at Law • 1972 – 1993)
Brooklyn Law School Brooklyn, New York
misongfoundation.org

CHAPTER 24: PREAMBLE TO OUR MISSION STATEMENT

A common thread that weaves corporations, charities, religions, and foundations, into one tapestry is that they all outline for themselves a goal or mission and then take the necessary steps to achieve that objective .We see ourselves somewhat differently.

We (the Mi Song Foundation) understand for example, that our goals (i.e. cancer confrontation and relief) are yet fully to be defined. Cancer succor will come, we believe, only through the optimal use of all available resources at any given time period. Strategy on the victim's behalf must be incremental and flexible.

Only tested relief options should be retained.

It may be said, therefore, that we in taking this journey are Pilgrims. Pilgrims in the sense that this is a new and uncharted course – yet one nonetheless filled with hope and optimism. It is a mission yet to define itself, but which cries out for a beginning.

And so, in honor of Mi Song, who before she died wanted very much to take this journey too, she (her Foundation) will take the first step and therefore this beginning. With God's blessing we will also succeed at it. misongfoundation.org

CHAPTER 25: WHAT WE DO

The Mi Song Foundation seeks to confirm or question cancer treatment effectiveness or value through Faith, education, and confrontation. This means, for example, that goals and improvement criteria are established (as a fluid ever changing modality) and these criteria are evaluated and retained or rejected as indicated pursuant to an ongoing review. This of course recognizes too that hospital, drug, or physician involvement in the client cancer struggle must be subject to an ongoing critical assessment.

It is, furthermore, the Foundation's belief that the success or failure of the cancer victim's struggle depends on large part in being able to use the Critical Review Process (described above) to identify and put to use those resources (hospital, doctors, drugs, etc.) which are optimal at any given time as the treatment phase moves from diagnosis to recovery. This means also that any critical resource evaluation must be fluid and ongoing. This will ensure that any resource not performing optimally will be modified or replaced. Recovery then will be more predictable.

Central to this philosophy is the recognition that the family unit must and is best able to engage as much as possible in the ongoing evaluation challenge. So too, it must be further said that resources must not be viewed as fixed or certain during the cancer treatment phase. If necessary, doctors or other modalities under review that fails to meet evaluation goals will be replaced or modified

to ensure that evaluation and treatment objectives
are being met.

CHAPTER 26: CONFRONTING CANCER

Cancer seeks no less than to take the life of an innocent victim. Although it seems obvious that all resources possible must be pressed into service to defeat this death threat, we believe that all too frequently effective confrontation is either not available or simply not identified.

We at The Mi Song Foundation begin with a discussion of who was Mia Song—i.e. what type of personality and influence—what, for example, can be learned from her struggle including her successes and her death. We then identify who in the victim's family is best able to perform those goal related functions more fully described at a later point in this brochure. We require that family members identify a team leader and create separate responsibility functions for doctor, hospital, chemotherapy, nursing, transportation, insurance and religious need effectiveness. It cannot be over emphasized that any evaluation of these modalities must be ongoing and critical.

Change in the acceptance or   continuation of any resource must be made whenever our standards are not met. If change is called for by the family protocol it must be done quickly.

Moreover, the Song Foundation believes that patient progress is not physician "centric"; Rather, whether a patient is showing adequate progress is a family/team evaluation after family performance criteria and resource result criteria (for example medical opinion) have been evaluated. Evaluation is recommended every 30 days or before each therapy session chemotherapy, radiation or doctor visit) whichever occurs first.

In addition, the importance of other possible healing or treatment systems, even when seen as non-traditional, must be considered. Holistic medicine is, or may be, quite useful in creating a successful recovery. This, most importantly includes prayer, faith and meditation.

The Mi Song Foundation believes that meditation, and the power of faith and trust in God are central and necessary for cancer survival and recovery.

This conviction is absolute and at the heart of the Mi Song message.

In the final analysis, the Song Mission sees as a primary importance—perhaps the only importance—the victims recovery, survival and well-being. Indeed, as long as cancer threatens, that danger invites and calls out for our rescue. This philosophy of care insists upon doctor, hospital and drug replacement or removal when called for under the protocol; that is, where performance goals or criteria are not being met. In this regard, the Mi Song Foundation will accept no deviation and will insist on taking an active part in all such change/replacement decisions. To state it again, this approach, rooted in the core beliefs of our Foundation, places patient or victim survival ahead of professional hubris or feelings, by insisting that physicians, hospital care, drug therapy etc. must and will be terminated and replaced if any fails to meet or exceed family/team performance criteria. This aggressive belief in God and method—indeed confrontational—defines us and is the living active spirit that moves our Foundation forward.

CHAPTER 27: WE QUESTION

An attempt must be made with no exception to verify and evaluate all statements, opinions, reports, and results etc, which relate to the victim's care and survival.

See and hear what you don't want to see and hear.

Do not see only what you want to see.

Authority sources are often wrong.

Question everything!

Verify if possible, what you see and are   told.

Nothing and no one is free from careful examination.

Ask questions! Question answers!

Good news may be the most dangerous!

Chances of survival increase as the victim identifies the "right" doctor, drug or hospital. Ask yourself: "How do I get there?" There may (and often are)   different paths. In the last analysis healing is in no small part, in your own hands. Doctors, hospitals and drugs are only aids to help the victim heal. Keep   control! Since victim recovery and well being are the only goals of the Mi Song Foundation.

We must also: Listen to the victim and learn what may not be obvious, i.e.; how does the victim rate his or her progress?   How about a victim's evaluation of the doctor, nurse, hospital and drug therapy experience?   How does the patient feel about money issues relating to their care? Progress, or perhaps a feeling by the patient of a lack of progress may not be evident.

Request that the patient evaluate and rate the Foundation protocol and protocol results. In addition, the patient's evaluation of family team performance must be obtained. The family responsibility in a life and death struggle requires not only the replacement and removal of professionals (physicians for example) but family team members as well when performance criteria are not being met.

CHAPTER 28: NEWS ACQUISITION AND DISSEMINATION (NAAD)

The Mi Song Foundation believes that patient/cancer victim treatment information must be managed carefully within the family involvement structure.

This approach will necessarily involve all of the following:

A family member will be designated under the working protocol to receive all patient information. Doctors, hospital staff and anyone involved in the patient's care must be advised that the family member so selected to receive patient news is exclusive and the only authorized news recipient. This family member will after total family review, provide the cancer victim with appropriate (that is news after family protocol review) information;

As stated above, the patient receives protocol family managed information only. Not all results need to be shared. For example, "bad" news is only made available to the patient after a family discussion after evaluation. The physician or hospital involvement must be advisory to the family and only through the designated family facilitator.

• All news received by the family unit must be tested against the Foundation protocol. No news ("good or bad") will be accepted for its accuracy or treatment value unless tested and verified. We have emphasized in our statement of mission that only God decides the success or failure of the patient's journey. This means that death must be resisted— i.e. not accepted by   patient or family, until such time as the Divine Will is made known. This does not mean that value based care (pain relieving drugs or hospice, for example) may not be of signif- icant use. However, since the   decision regarding the victim's death or recovery lies with the Creator the role of hospice care must be life directed. Hos- pice as an adjunct or of palliative use to the vic- tim's recovery is welcome. We must recognize how- ever that there are many examples of patients who have had vigor restored when hope for recovery seemed all but lost. Finally it is our conviction that cancer success requires us to believe that death or defeat is never acceptable. Cancer treatment deci- sions must not be based upon its inevitability. Death or   recovery is written upon the palm of the Divine Will. The ultimate outcome only resides there. Any opinion, medical or otherwise, which at- tempts to predict the futility of ongoing, continu- ous, aggressive treatment that is life directed and hopeful, must and will be rejected.

CHAPTER 29: THE ROLE OF GOD ROOTED IN THE MI SONG FOUNDATION

Mi Song endured anguish, depression, pain, doubt, failure, heartbreak and finally death and all during a torture filled cancer struggle. She nonetheless, stayed hopeful and sanguine. She believed, and often discussed with me, for example, that in the universe her destiny was safe and in the ever care of a divine, loving Creator—a spiritual force (and she never failed to smile as she would tell this to me) both kind and benevolent and, more importantly, one who cared about all life – including of course, hers. We laughed often about Woody Allen's view of death: "I'm not afraid to die," said Allen, "As long as I'm not there when it happens."

Mi Song too was unafraid to die. She believed that her Creator would take her at death and keep her safe for eternity. She was absolutely sure there is a special destiny for each of us. Her Foundation now sends this message: "Hope and faith in the benevolent will of our divine Creator, a will that requires for the victim of cancer only what is ultimately good and best for that victim, is the only way to recovery and the realization of God's Plan."

In summary, our views indeed confrontational may seem harsh or offensive to some. We question all human based authority and test, where possible, everything. But, we believe also that in the final analysis this is the best course. Could Mi Song have lived if we had followed this path more faithfully during her cancer filled struggle? We will never know; but what this memory conscious Foundation does know, and I surely know is that only she was she.

She will never exist again.

Her death had now come.

It was the day,
indeed that terrible day,

"The day the music died."

REFERENCES

U.S. News and World Report

Health Med.com

Qualitycheck.org

Hosptalcompare.com

Consumer Reports Health.com

Safe Patient Project.org

Leapfroggroup.org

Rwif.org

U.S. Oncology.com

Neverevents.org

Health Watch USA

MyCancerNews.com

RobertsRcview.com

- Doctors and hospitals kill by negligence over 200,000 Americans each year! More than any U.S. war.
- Drug companies pay doctors to give patients drugs that are more expensive but less effective.
- Doctors use hospice to fleece you and Medicare.
- If your doctor is an atheist, your death is more likely.

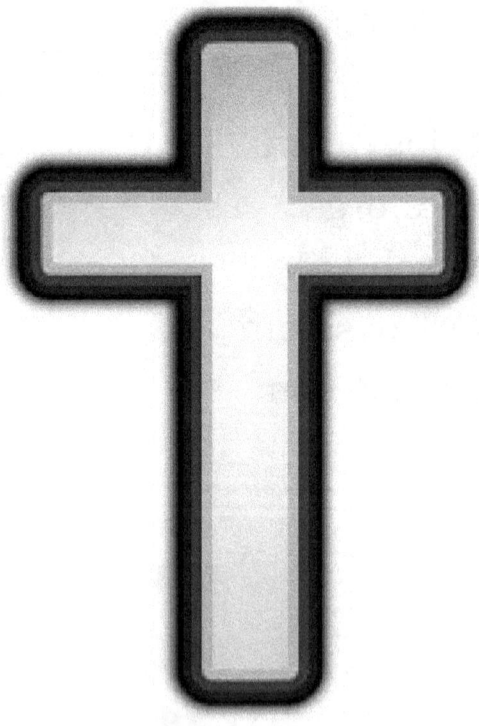